# Topical Anesthesia

Perspectives on Medicine and Life

H. Wesley Brown M. D.

Pantoum Press
Painesville, Ohio

Published by Pantoum Press, P.O. Box 362, Painesville, Ohio 44077

Printed in United States of America

Cover design and drawings by Kim Oswald

Library of Congress Catalog Card Number:  99-93227

ISBN  0-9671627-0-X

Acknowledgement

Reprinted by Permission of the publishers and the Trustees of Amherst College from  THE POEMS OF EMILY DICKINSON, Thomas H. Johnson, ed. , Cambridge, Mass,: The Belknap Press of Harvard University Press, Copyright © 1951, 1955, 1979, 1983 by the President and Fellows of Harvard College.

*for*
*Eric and Lydia*

*contents*

*contents*

Surgeons must be very careful

When they take the knife!

Underneath their fine incisions

Stirs the Culprit - *Life*!


Emily Dickinson

# *Preface*

One embarks upon any journey with a certain degree of eagerness and anxiety.  So it was with the decision to prepare the following pages for publication.

Many of these poems have seen the light of day in hospital newsletters, newslike weeklies and , on occasion, a wider audience.  Others have merely been presented to my friends at the Poets League of Greater Cleveland Workshiop.  The remainder have resided only in my head or  computer until this time.

As  will become obvious with the readings of the poems, they were written at different times of my life.  A number were written quite a few years ago and several most recently. It is surprising that my thoughts on certain subjects still seem valid and/or appropriate to the present day.

The decision to include both non-medical and non-humorous material (the reader, of course, is entitled to make this distinction) was based on a belief that broader subjects are at least tangential to the larger experience (see E. Dickinson poem).

Medicine is, has always been, a challenging profession. Some of the challenges have been eliminated while others have taken their place. The newer ones involve fewer "blood and guts" issues and more cerebral ones ( CME, liability of all kinds economics, ets.) but still must be dealt with if doctors are to continue to save lives and inprove the well-being of their patients. The front cover nothwithstanding, doctors will always put their patients first and other considerations secondary.

I want to thank in particular the writers and poets who have offered encouragement, criticism, editing and coaching in the preparation of this manuscript, specifically Cyril Dostal, Jill Sell, Kat Blackbird, Pam and Chuck McGuire and again, the members of the Poets League of Greater Cleveland Workshop.

In closing, it is my wish that you enjoy these poems, have a few good laughs (or chuckles or even smiles as the case may be) and live your lives with at least some of the irrepressible exhuberance that my patients exhibit and bring to mine.

H. W. B.

# 1 The Patient's Perspective

Dad:   Tell me son,
        what's the worst disease
        in the world?
Son (2nd year medical student):
        Really can't say dad, there are
        a lot of pretty bad ones...I give up,
        you tell me.
Dad:   The one that gets you.

# INJECTION!

Now comes the night nurse perusing my chart,
smiling that smile and pushing her cart,
her name is Brunhilde and quite overfed,
as she states with a winking
"It's time for your med."


"Just wait a sec," I implore in a flash,
"Put away your sharp things, don't do anything rash.
There is room for discussion in matters  as these,
maybe treatment less radical for my disease.


My bowels are stirring,  my fever's at bay,
I have a new dartboard if you'd care to play,
What's wrong  with you anyway, childhood off track?
Why needle me now for whatever you lack?


My doctor had hinted he'd switch me to pills,
if the emeses ended and ditto the chills.
He's on call tonight, right at home, by the phone,
on the edge of his chair, waiting there, all alone."

She senses my fear, but cares not a whit,
enjoying it even, I'm sure she'd admit.
She closes the door and grabs her syringe,
while I disappear undercover and cringe,


Will my plea be pointless, or could she now pause,
and take from the Tubex  her drawing of "JAWS?"
No way will it happen, she's strong, sure and fast,
with her piercing insult as I had forecast.


Excuses are useless,  my fate's in her hands,
a prayer and a squirm my last song and dance,
her spot not too far from my midline crevasse,
she probably thinks I'm a pain in the...neck.

Orthopedic Nurse

We agree there's a lot to be said

for a pretty young nurse near your bed,

but forget the action when strung up in traction

and just send an old one instead.

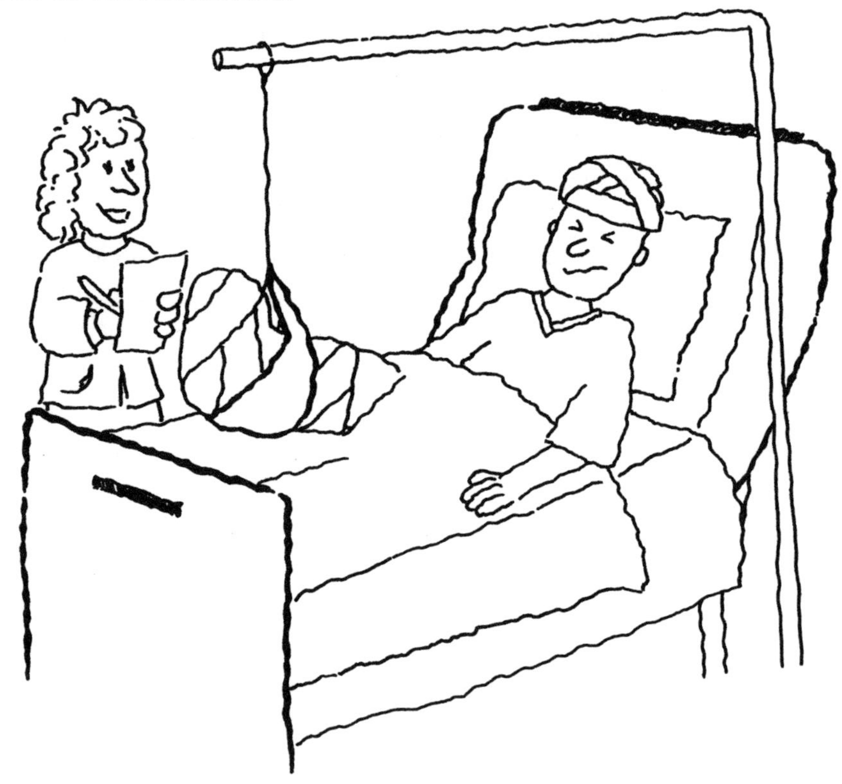

4

# MIOK?

Admitted just for tests,
I had hoped for "R & R,"
but q2h they took my B.P.
and my T. P.R.

The first night I was visited
by M.O.M. h.s.,
how glad I was for BRP,
my bowel's last request.

That a.m. I was NPO
before my GTT,
I drank my breakfast cola stat,
then had an MI p.c.

I t was PDQ to the SCU
to run my EKG,
they wired me to a TV screen
and cancelled my B.E.

Then came an IV ASAP
dripping D5 and NS.
a  CVP was inside of me
as the lido came on express.

Stable now, my VS normal,
but enter the lovely nurse Nell,
One whole body scan and the trouble began,
as my heart played a rhythm from Hell.

Pounding and jumping, my PMI thumping,
I threw some PVCs,
Was I going to arrest while fully undressed?
Where were my BVDs?

Yet we slipped back into NSR
as I had a change of heart,
Then Nell took my pulse at the femoral site
and they grabbed the defib from the cart.

Zap!! Three hundred joules coursed through my chest,
again I was converted,
"Wow," I bemused, "a most drastic way
to have your libido diverted."

Recovering fast, my next few days
were bitter pills to swallow,
expecting Venus in cap of white,
I looked up and saw Apollo.

No more TLC, PRN or SAP,
would come from Nell and her nurses,
creating DOE, SOB in frail me
from bellowing assorted curses.

Oh, somewhere in this place of ill
the days are short and easy,
and somewhere still, when the patient's a pill,
he's not made to feel so queasy.

Though some may eat and some may drink
to excess when stresses climb,
there will always be those who try to compose
and turn their vices to rhyme.




Medical abbreviations: in order of appearance,
q2h (every two hours),
B.P.(blood pressure),
T.P.R. (temperature, pulse, respiratory rate),
MOM (milk of magnesia),
h.s. (hour of sleep, " hora somni"),
BRP (bathroom privileges),
NPO (nothing by mouth, "per os"),
GTT  (glucose tolerance test),
MI (myocardial infarction),
p.c. ( after meals),

PDQ (pretty da-- quick),

SCU (special care unit- shouldn't every unit give "special car

EKG (electrocardiogram),

B.E. (barium enema),

IV (intravenous),

D5,NS (dextrose - 5%, Normal saline),

CVP (central venous placement),

PMI (point of maximal intensity),

PVC (premature ventricular contraction),

NSR (normal sinus rhythm),

TLC (tender loving care),

prn (as necessary),

SAP (soon as possible),

DOE (dyspnea on exertion),

SOB (shortness of breath),

stat (immediately)

The Lab

A myriad of tests to provide the right clue,

to aid and abet your veiled diagnosis.

If we order enough maybe one is askew,

but could be your same old neurosis.

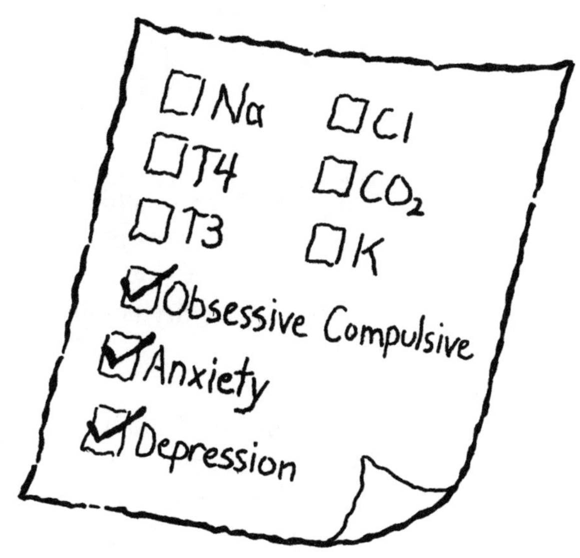

True Blue Flu


About once a year
with hardly a sound,
when you least expect trouble
the flu comes around.


And we who are bitten
can't pick up the phone,
no working, no playing,
we're sick to the bone.


At first there's a chill
as the fever takes off,
then the scratchy raw throat
and the brassy dry cough.


In a matter of  hours
you're home and in bed,
and listening to strains
of some old Grateful Dead.


You cough and you vomit,
and don't bat an eye,
like a wrung - out old dishrag
that's hung out to dry.

Whoever had said that
it lasts but a day,
was just spreading the lie
of a hopeful cliché.


The truth of the matter
sans shadow of doubt
is that flu lasts a week
hanging on - dragging out.


A tiny voice whispers
from inside my spleen,
"Come next fall (if we're out of bed),
GET THE VACCINE!!

My Dental Visit

(or, have I got a Cavitron for you)


I guess it had been awhile (so maybe it was a few years)
 since I visited my dentist who worked in the same building
(was proximity to blame?)
and again conquered my oral anxiety,
 though I generally strayed far and wide
from the tooth and gum game.


And even though it my afternoon was free and my agenda,
though empty, could easily have been filled (unlike my teeth),
I stopped by anyway and she said
she would "fit me in," her face aglow,
and though I assured her I could come back another day
if it would be better, etc.,
she more or less insisted...............soooo....

There I was, sitting in the new "comfortable contoured chair,"

staring blankly out the window,

greeting my hygienist Kim with my defective smile

and blubbering innocuous patter,

as she chastised me for no-shows, took X-rays,

said something like "OH,MY!!"

and quickly got to the nitty-gritty, mostly the latter.


I told her it was my fault (I had a bad attitude-

I leave my teeth alone, they leave me alone)

and she began to lecture.

Now Kim is cute (though the effect is muted with her mask on),

but the song and dance of the dental hygienist

was familiar to me and while I don't listen well,

I could conjecture.

So I opened my mouth and one of those

ten-foot long grappling hooks entered my stoma,

and then began the scraping, the picking,

the squirting and choking which

should only be done when one is in coma.


"C'mon, " I remonstrated, "don't be a wimp,"

lying there simpering like a toothless invertebrate

(which was the life form I preferred extantly)

as she slipped along from fang to tusk

using methods nefarious.

But she had shifted into a serious kind of rhythm

(no, not that kind)  and from time to time

I would fantasize (fun in the sun, anyone?)

until she made a mistake (just kidding, Kim)

and touched one of my "sensitive areas."

Attempting to converse

(a nervous energy release kind of thing)

was futile as she toiled on

with a relentless focused fury,

and as I grunted she would say,

"Just a few more" and I could only

hold my tongue (get the picture?)

 as if to say, "What, me worry?"


But at last she completed her exploratory surgery

and began polishing with her "crunchy style" toothpaste

 and dental "Moto-Tool,"

swooping and swerving around my oral cavity

like a swallow heading south,

and again I felt like a "ninety pound weakling"

who gets sand thrown into his face (and mouth).

But I rinsed for the final time (there is a God!)

 and thought I was through,

when OUT OF NOWHERE she grabs this THING

 and says,"Have I got a CAVITRON for you!"


"Oh no you don't," I'm thinking

as she slams me back into "The Chair"

and begins zapping me with her "laser,"

so what if it was just a high-tech low-sodium bicarb squirter,

my protests wouldn't faze her.


Then at last my favorite dentist arrived

and confirmed that WE

had a few problems WE could fix,

and asked me to make an appointment on the way out

and WE could fill them in an afternoon, all SIX!

And I really would have done so,

but I had to check my schedule

and call them back which I will do

 as soon as I can find that silly thing,

but I really should show you my bright shiny teeth,

glistening and a good deal whiter than customary,

all the tiny irregularities notwithstanding.


And anyway the whole experience deserves a good rhyme,

'Cause you never can tell

 (maybe I put my schedule over there...no...

over here...no...I haven't the foggiest idea...)

when there'll be a next  time.

## Hospital Discharge Planner

Too long you've been here, but want to stay longer,
    have taken death's holiday twice;
then soon you will meet with our sweet Discharge Planner,
    the one who will tell you "No Dice."

She's heard every excuse you can find in the book
    (and many that aren't even there),
from "just one more day" to "insurance will cover,"
    and  "I have no clean underwear."

From "still have this cough" to "my daughter works days,"
    and "I'm getting on in my years,"
no matter how gory  your "I can't go" story,
    the whole thing will fall on deaf ears.

There she goes again now, shaking the beds,
    as fast as admitting can fill 'em,
if fever results from this quick readjustment,
    our Billing Department will chill 'em.

# 2    *The Doctor's Perspective*

*Laughter is ...*
*the Music of Life*
William Osler

On Accepting Ones's Lot in Life

It's really no hardship at all
and we're not handicapped as a rule,
but you walk twice as far at the mall,
and a few more steps makes one no fool.


But whatever the cause or the basis,
(since there's really no need to displace us),
we request, in your lot,
please park in your spot,
and stop taking up doctor's spaces.

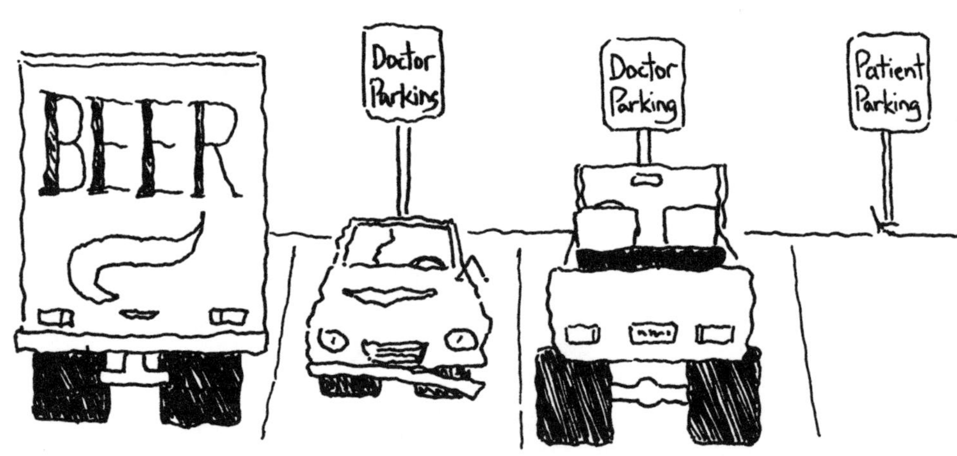

## Intern ER Soliloquy

Soon or late, rough but ready, I'm eager to see,
a bonafide sick-as-hell  emergency,
some moribund who cries out - Intervention!
(an illness or trauma too ghastly to mention.)

Forget the toenails and day-old  cephalgia,
take back your backaches, neuritis, neuralgia,
bring on the blood, the guts and the gore!
still I wait  'cause the big stuff's the resident's chore.

Oh, once in a while they ask my assistance,
to hold someone down if they give some resistance,
I know the routine cases, bring me some action!
a bad DKA or a bone that wants traction.

But come three a.m., I'm first to the foray,
a life on the line in my territory,
Residents sleep ( how they hate to arise),
Suggestions? A few, and most "ill" advised.

As the morning arrives I shall bid fond adieu,
till my next turn on call at our ghoulish drive-thru,
learning the things that I'll need down the line,
awaiting the day when the patient's all mine.

The Beeper

"Hang onto your seats, boys, it's going to be a bumpy ride."  Bette Davis
  With apologies to S. Coleridge and the Mystery Science Fiction Theatre


He was a beeper bearer,
though silent at this time,
but his tale shall be told and please, don't scold
'cause it's all comin' down in sweet rhyme.   <sub>"get the dramamine, Captain,
                                                I feel an emesis coming on"...</sub>


The song a sleepless sorrow,
but life's an honest school,
the beeper bearer finds fate no fairer,
yet  now he plays the fool.                    ...or was it the bassoon...


For no one loves the beeper
yet no one dares to tell,
the Devil's best friend going off without end,
making a sound straight from hell.    ...kind of an aural Chinese water torture


It startles you while driving,
and jostles your digestion,
right on your hip
in misplaced comradeship,
just waiting to make a suggestion.    .."they need you in OB stat, Doctor"...


At "the Game," with cards, or on "the throne,"
loudly it would chime,
no sense of discretion, just simple oppression,
and never a call at halftime.                ...and  I had a straight flush...

22

When I was just a student,
living  laissez-faire,
it was only my heart and illegible chart
that one brought to intensive care.   ...well, maybe some cheeze whiz and crackers...


But internship awaited me,
and so my nickel and dime,
enforced servitude  in the guise of  Joe Screwed
and a beeper that worked overtime.          ...wow, it's playing Phillip Glass...


Residency was better,
a raise and some respect,
but not from the box  of squeaks and squawks,
a condition none could correct.          ...if it's prison, how 'bout a cell phone


Things started to get better as
 I dreamed of life in Boise,
 but fall off to sleep and it'd go beep ,
 'cause all it knew was noisy.                ...and I'm getting woisey...

Then on to private practice
to get some peace and quiet,
but the answering service was too nervous quervous,
so I took out a room at the Hyatt.        ..error, ambulance driver scared lobbyists...

Into the woods my love and I
might now be left alone,
though we were enticed, our ardor was iced,
when the darn thing went off on its own.          ...Lovus interruptus...


There was a time its simple tone
called forth the bright and brave;
to be summoned this way, it seemed to say,
you had a life to save.          ...ala Casey, Kildare, Welby, Benton
                                 and Hands-on-Harry at Preschool.


Now pizza drivers have them,
and crossing guards and such,
whatever info, you gotta have mo,
and it's never  too fast or too much.     ..."this is Maple and Elm, we have
                                          a J-walker in custody, 2nd grade".....


Unlike the ancient  mariner,
who needed no Blue Cross,
my HMO says take it and go,
it's your personal albatross.          ...Like, go where??, and Volare to you too...


Yesterday at breakfast,
while rapidly chewing my Chex,
it went off and I choked, gasped and croaked,
amidst other special effects.          ...you don'wanna know...

At first I felt frustration,
but then it was anger and hate,
so I picked up the box  with the zinger,
and flung it to its fate.                    ...had it coming..


No longer will it taunt me,
with screechings at noon-tide;
another bare doc in beeper battered shock,
wanders the countryside.              … and makes house calls...

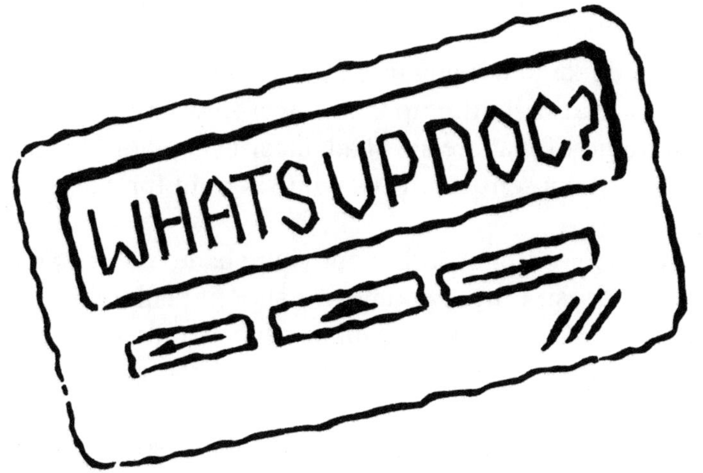

# The Chromology of Rhinorrhea

If you wake with runny nose and you itch to diagnose,
do not fret about the color of the ooze.
When a sneeze or big kerchoo leaves an unfamiliar hue,
such as sky-blue pink, vermillion or chartreuse.

For the cause of nasal drip which is on your fingertip
is no riddle that is far beyond your ken.
And the answer to be found is not by color bound,
nor written in some ancient book of Zen.

'Cause I'd like to tell you true , there's no research in full view
that will offer up the answer to your query.
Just no proof that green is bad, clear is good or blue is sad,
yet consensus tells us white is right for dairy.

So do not fret or fuss 'bout your shade of mucopus,
doesn't mean you need a shot of penicillin.
Buy some Kleenex, get a hanky; whatever, don't be cranky,
blame it on the nasty virus - it's the villain.

Now the truth you have in hand , do not blame some obscure gland,
get some chicken soup and serve it piping hot.
Just don't wax debilitate, at this nasal Watergate,
I can't say it any clearer when it'snot.

## Record Room Lament ( Dear Doctor,....)

Are your H.& P.'s done?
Are your summaries complete?
Did you dictate today?
Did you sign the front sheet?

If your answer is yes,
then you've been a good doc,
and you won't find your head
on the old chopping block.

But if not I'd make rounds incognito,
and watch for the chair and the whip,
for it's part of the MRT credo,
not to let the docs out of their grip.

For these ladies are tougher than tough,
they chew nails, eat raw eggs and stuff.
So the very next time they suggest that you sign,
do it fast or they just might get rough.

'cause I once knew a doc from Lakeshore,
whose "INCOMPLETE"'s  were 'to die for,'
Well, they found him in parts, buried under his charts,
so whose job is it NOW, por favor?

Cheap Miracles

A long time ago when you just didn't know
who you should ask or where you could go,
You could call on old doc, 'cause he'd been to school,
and he learned everything, while you're playing pool.

But today you don't sweat, we have info galore,
talkin' medical stuff from ceiling to floor,
from home health advisors to on-line Brittanicas,
pharmacy handouts and obscure botanicas.

You can ask Dr. Donahue, Abby or Ann,
or maybe that ad from chiropractor Dan,
and 'zines like "Today's Health," "Prevention" and such,
a lot of advice and you don't pay too much.

Plus a lot of docs pay the paper to print
a column or two to provide a "health  hint,"
you won't look too far for an "ailment du jour,"
on the latest disease and a miserly cure.

Did I mention your friend's or relative's potion,
a substance more likely to launch undue motion?
No matter that doc might still have an edge,
on matters of  health, you're not out on a ledge.

Both  grandmas are locked into knowledge of Spock
and Brazelton too--does that come as a shock?
Every nursery school marm will tell you "informal,"
of your "hyper" pre-schooler that you thought was normal.

Have I mentioned the para-professionals "x",
the physician's assistants, the aides and the techs,
and nurse practictioners of all descriptions
who gladly write all your needed prescriptions?

Is the answer you seek still outside your grasp?
Perhaps the psychologist is one to ask,
Or maybe a teacher, a minister, lawyer,
the bartender right down the street, or Tom Sawyer?

When all's said and done, what say - you're confused?
And feel that you suffer from knowledge abused?
I hate to say it but we're not amused,
Why not call 'ol  doc, what have you to lose?

# URI

Could it be a Russian spy,
or the acronym from Hell,
Unclaimed Ransoms of Ionia,
Unknown Rappers of Intel?

Could have gone with MND*,
ARU** or SRN***,
more objective to be sure,
not a diagnostic fen.

We all grew fond of YUB,
CMP and BLT.
So why not URU?
Could we live with IME?


*mucoid nasal discharge
**acute rhinorrhea, unspecified
***simple runny nose

CME #1

Once in a while  I do enjoy a colleague's talk,
a new idea, a new technique, a little chalk,
a safer drug, a rare disease and better tools,
all reasons to excite the brain beyond the rules.

But now too often all is just rehash,
or two weeks later than a late news flash,
but still I'll go (the law says so)  and persevere,
for painful loss of cash and time, it's in one ear.

CME  #2
 (Are they serving lunch?)

It's time to go fishing for CME,
in Hawaii, Chicago or old N.Y.C.,
I'll bait my hook with plenty of green,
and hide in the back row, sight unseen,

'Till a really big "fish" rises fast and strikes,
grabbing my lure (the color he likes).
I'll let him run and tire himself out,
but he's pretty long winded, leaving doubt.

At last in the net, we put him on ice,
and thank him for making this small "sacrifice."
Now he's safe in my fridge for the auditing crew,
'cause you can't have your credits and eat them too.

## Homo erectus*

We have a new drug that is not a soft sell,
sildenafil citrate but don't kiss and tell,
A tiny trick tonic to take up the slack,
forget little sheldon, Big Joe has come back!

A baby blue tablet with power sublime,
a chemical spell when you're playing for time,
at last the long pipeline has yielded some fruit;
it helps if your pockets are loaded with loot.

But first we should check out what's under your pate,
perhaps a psychiatrist might set you straight?
Said he, " If you check out my soft interlink,
you'll see why the last thing I want is a shrink.

Remember the days when tumescence was sure,
no one disappointed, it was its own cure,
But now it's a dangler and not the Grand Prix,
he's out of a job passing time and sweet pee."

But wait, not to worry; your ship has come in,
your mast will be straighter than it's ever been,
You'll sail 'round the world, just ask good old doc,
"Is it true 'bout niagra - or just poppycock?"


*This poem can easily be sung to "sweet Betsy from Pike"

# Discharge

Once should be enough of this signing out stuff,
   "Home Today" and just sign your name,
 but it's "no way  Jose " in the Record Room way,
   as we play the Complete-the-Chart game.


First the Progress Note sheet (better find a good seat)
   what you write here is just the beginning,
Be sure to write clearly or you will pay dearly
   to those who are right now just grinning


And picking your charts and finding again
   the evil undotted 'i,'
and spending a blue moon scanning each page,
   (could this be their natural high?).


Still nothing's complete! Where's the Summary sheet?
   of  my patient's quick stop in this place.
So it was a short stay - let's call it a day -
   Fill it out!  It's their new data base.

Try to make some quick rounds, do your discharge exam,
    (talk to patients??),  be fast and record it,
Be sure to report (this could end up in court),
    all details straight and true, not distorted.


We're nearing the end, to the Face Sheet attend,
    and list every malady codable,
Every twitch, every turn, every off-hand concern,
    it's alright if they're not so notable.


We're getting close now - there's the old checkered flag,
    call it done - Fini - you're in clover!
But Wait!! (it's so late),  No!! Not the Wrong DATE!!
    What was that you said? Do it OVER?

# 3 The Pediatric Perspective - Both Sides

"the child is father of the man,
but not for quite a while,..."

Ogden Nash

## Lamaze

"This is a baby," is how we begin,
as we try to prepare for the little urchin.
Soon to be born and lo...there's the rub,
You won't be ready when he needs a scrub.


No matter how many books you have read,
child psych courses taken or neighbor's kid's fed,
It'll be different when "johnny comes home,"
and starts to cry out like a sick metronome.


Your faces so eager to hear all the "scoop,"
will change just a bit with the first sign of "poop."
But you'll 'pick it up' as you go along,
and baby will tell you when you've got it wrong.


We talk about feeding, jaundice and colic,
cord care and 'spitting up' add to the frolic;
All about vitamins, water and sleep,
and crying all night (will get you in deep).

The slide show spectacular brings little comfort,
as onto the screen giant babies cavort;
X-rated and blue, squish-squashed and twisted,
sights you had hardly imagined existed.


The formal talk ended, why are you so pale?
There won't be a test on every detail.
"Don't worry," I tell them, "Just do your best,
and anyway it's a bit late to protest."


We open it up for"any old questions,"
as "this may be dumb..." and "what of congestion."
No one can guess what a new mom will ask,
Mistakenly, you think you're up to the task.


It's " My grandma says...and she raised twenty four,"
I reply, " But we just don't do that anymore."
Eyes roll up. Check the clock! My how time flies!
As you leave, don't glance back, at the terror in their eyes!

Discrimination

I 'm just a yellow baby,
you had two yesterday,
and more of us tomorrow,
we just won't go away.

We are not tickled pink at all
to have this saffron hue,
my liver cuts in *manana,*
yet my heels are black and blue.

Not easy being yellow,
before you've learned to crawl,
picking a sleeper just my shade
for a first trip to the mall.

I could be Asian sweetness
but mama says I'm not,
the apple of  my Daddy's eye,
or was it apricot?

Here I'm pink, there I'm blue,
blending with the yellow.
Match me up with Rainbow Brite,
I'm a lucky fellow.

A new face, it's the lab girl,
all tubes and sharp her lance,
she's makin'me cry and lookit
what I just did in my pants.

Go right ahead and stick me,
but not the box with lights;
too much stimulation and then deprivation,
my senses will never be right.

So bring on the fiberlights bright,
I'll be pink as a rose in bloom,
but what's the deal with this mooey-meal,
not mother's best I presume?

How long will I be stuck here?
Send me home, let's cut to the quick;
septic I'm not, you know it,
just mellow yellow and  homesick.

# Hospital Nursery

Silent and still
(save the fussy one by the window)
the brave, the unassuming
even for a shrinking planet their shoulders too tiny
ready to consume, complain and consecrate
no cold feet about global warming
no discontent (at this moment)
deliberating destiny
basking in the world's goodness
the not-yet-prime-time-players,
saviours of the millenium
wait patiently
(save the fussy one by the window)

# Double Check-up

Andrew and Michael were two years and four,
classic male sibling rivals on opening the door,
The room all at once seemed a trifle too small,
then bigger as Andy shoved Mike down the hall.


Mike would have none of this , fur started flying,
as  Mom stood by Andy and Mike started crying.
I closed the door quickly and greeted the mother,
whose disheartened face seemed to lip sync, "Oh brother!"


The eldest was first, not at all full of fear,
as he yanked at the stethescope still in my ear.
I winced and he laughed, then screamed in the bell,
a noise that I knew was a sound straight from Hell.


I tried for too long to examine his belly,
which shook when he laughed  'cause my hands were "too chilly."
A gonadal check he was quick to decline,
I concurred when a fast knee was slammed into mine.


His gait seemed OK as he ran down the hall,
but he wouldn't come back to the room, I recall.
It was on to the two-year old , Andy by name,
but he wanted no part of my "physical game."

He clung to his Mom with the strength of a Titan,
and clearly was well into kickin' and fightin',
(not to mention bitin').
Introductions were skipped, we proceded informal,
from what I could hear, his heart seemed quite normal.

His ears he preferred to be left all alone,
but we took a quick peek and his voice raised a tone.
Moving along I checked out his throat,
as his subsequent emesis streamed down my coat.

His lungs he exercised sans intermission,
from his now tightly wound and coiled fetal position,
We talked about toileting, Mom said, "No Way!"
I agreed that it still might wait one more day.

She had a few questions which took half a hour,
and quickly I sensed that both needed a shower,
But finally finished I filled out the forms,
and reassured Mom that her boys fit the norms.

Though  hearing's now normal and body not blue,
I still shake a little and swallow hard,
( and a chill goes up my spine)
when I enter a room
for a check-up times two.

# Perspective

Why can't you be serious child,
don't you know the world is wild?
Chase that grin and run it down,
this is no age for a clown.

Not to criticize your style,
but planet earth is now on trial,
Listen, look and feel the pain,
then announce we're not insane.

One might think you just don't care,
with your tousled unkempt hair,
Still it seems that life smiles back,
loving the laughing face you wear.

# Growing Up

is not age, pounds or inches,
but getting through the clinches,
not tables of multiplication,
but fables of felicitation.


Not 1st place, all A's or the Prom,
but separating from Mom,
being left off the team,
or losing a dream.


Time for opening the eyes and  heart,
looking inside,
taking apart,
accepting  all, nothing denied,
making  changes, becoming
what (we think) we want to be,
in dysrythmic drumming.

Time for looking outside,
logging onto www dot cosmos,
choosing right, left, or wrong, but wide-eyed,
judging, trusting yourself (not  MS - DOS),
Deciding what  you want to keep
(doesn't mean you get to keep it)
and what to throw on the junkheap,
your psychic retrofit.


Considering what options
to leave in the drawer,
affirming errors,
moving on,
making more.

palivizumab


If you're just a tiny baby with a bias bent to wheeze,
and apprehension lingers over RSV disease,
There is monoclonal magic poppin' fresh out of the lab,
with a name that's hoot'n holler, it's called palivizumab.

It's a "pal" for "viz"ing babes, as it "zum"s into the  blood,
With those killer antibodies, it's a philanthropic scud,
By injection once a month 'till the weather's not so drab,
stay at home and off the ward with some palivizumab.

## Neo-Freudian

I had just checked the newborn and was preparing to leave the exam room when the three year-old sibling came up to me and asked, " Is Alligator Breath ok? " I looked quizzically at the parents who returned my puzzled countenance.

In a second they had exchanged glances and began laughing. I joined in shortly after a second peek at the chart recalled the baby's name, "Abigail Beth."

Exam

The boy was five years old and I had just concluded
my complete preschool examination which included "private parts."
He retired to the corner of the room and dressed while I talked
 to his mother about kindergarten.  I was at the door ready to exit
when he walked right up to me, red-faced, and announced
quite seriously, "Next time, I'm going to check yours."

Appearances

When I was in solo practice my vacations were infrequent. During one particular absence I had decided to grow  a mustache and beard which would be at least presentable on my return.  My first day back, one mother commented to her son, "Doesn't Dr. Brown look different?"  The four year-old took a good look, thought a few seconds and asked, " Doctor, Did you take a bath?"

# 4  Limeritis

*No matter how grouchy you're feeling,*
*You'll find that a limerick is healing,*
*It grows in a wreath*
*all around the front teeth,*
*Thus preventing the face from congealing.*

*anon.*

A urologist from Santee,
worked in an ocean of pee,
The money he made!
in the name of free trade!
But would anyone do it for free?


A nurse from hot Escondido,
would dance on a pole at the Lido,
her charms on display
moved every which way,
which we all thought was well, pretty neat-o.


A hospital administrator,
coming straight from Decatur,
bought a giant balloon
(but she fell in a swoon
and burst as he tried to inflate her).

A lawyer who followed disaster,
at which he was truly past master,
pursued too close and fast
and would up in a cast,
so we had to waste four pounds of plaster.


A surgeon from quiet DesMoines,
such an expert at things in the groin,
if there was a doubt,
he would just cut it out,
and close with tincture of benzoin.


A records tech from L.A.,
went for a roll in the hay,
but there was no teasin'
because of her wheezin'
and nothing to write here today.

# 5 The Meteorologic Perspective

*"There will be a 50% chance*

*of snow showers today."*

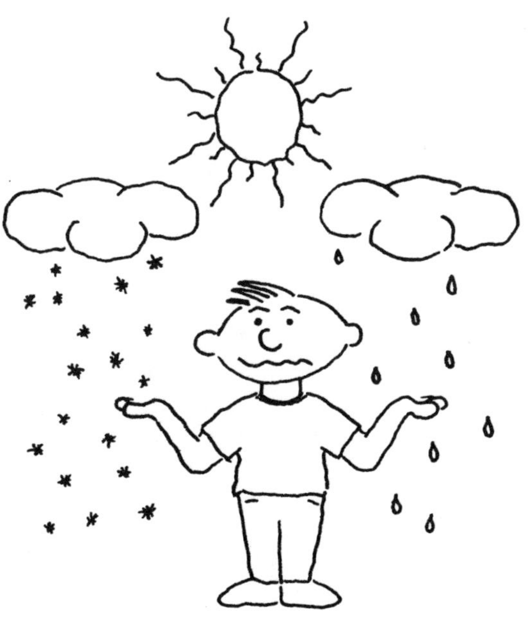

# Snow

Some like it thick and wet, some powder dry,
Some like it piled up as high as the sky,

Some like it draped over nature's fair bowers,
Some like it better than spring's  gentle showers,

Some like to just watch it drift past their shutters,
Some like it melted, down in the gutters.

Raindrops

Maybe God was weeping

as He played his Creation game,

Maybe He said after snowflakes,

"This is too much trouble,

let's make them all the same."

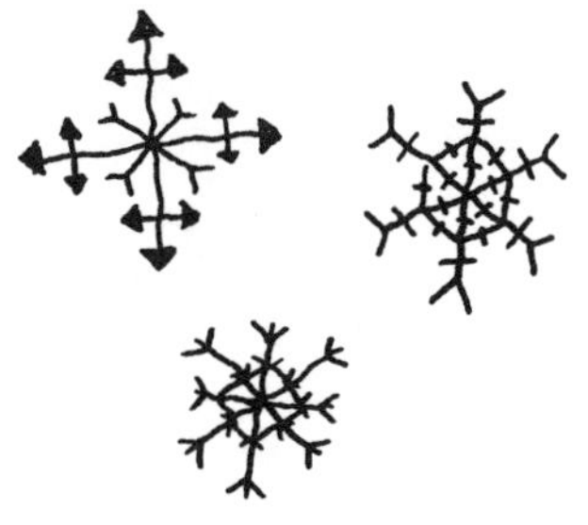

# 6  *The Communicator's Perspective*

*The Medium is the Message*

*Marshall McLuhan*

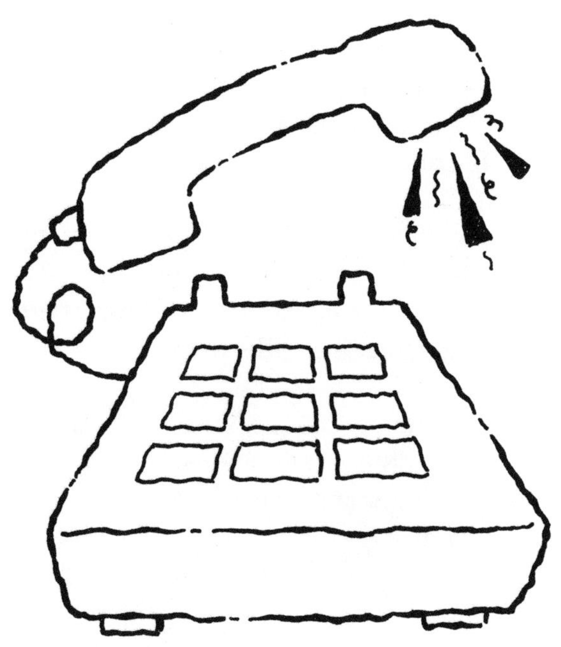

No, you may not


"Can I put you on hold ,"she said with a smile,
"for just a few seconds and not a long while?"
before I could answer, someone's selling cars,
and singing "America," (just a few bars);

Right after they chimed in with music of Bach,
followed by Mozart, as I checked the clock;
but along came a new voice with,"You're next in line!"
a short pause to find it's just  me on the vine,

I got some more music, enticing to stay,
but my hair's growing longer and now it looks gray,
Then along came a news report-floods, flu and fires,
did she say "a few seconds,"  I'm talking to Liars!!!

Next came a third voice with a menu so long,
that I feared to choose any lest one get it wrong;
It was "Press one for touch tone phone, press two for CIA,
press three for silly songs, press four  to waste away,"

But then, from the Void, came the very First Voice,
with a tone so delicious, she left me no choice,
So gentle and sweet was her "Are you still there?"
that my first thought was "Gee - then you do <u>truly care</u>."

A short silence followed, but not like before,
now gleeful and sure that I'd  pass through her door,
"I'll connect you right now," is just what she said,
and all I recall is a line that went dead.

# Doodle Oodle

Warble warble goes the phone,
like the theme from "Twilight Zone,"
less annoying by a hair,
than a case of mal de mer.

Such a noise is not a treat,
not unlike a thrush in heat,
like a larynx in a sling,
makes one wish for ding-a-ling.

# 7    *Circumspective*

*Laughter is a tranquilizer with no side effects.*

Arnold Glasow

Leaves  of  Lawn

Soft yet resilient, clean and upright,
the color you love at the traffic light,
belated praise surely, but let's raise a glass,
Give three cheers for fescue, let's hear it for grass.

Imagine a world of concrete and dirt,
ugly and painful, you fall and get hurt.
We take for granted the good earth's softwear,
what's thought to be meadow is really green hair.

Without it your golf game drops in a hole,
soccer and baseball folks give up and bowl.
Don't give me Astroturf, gimme a break,
of maybe an arm or a leg, for Pete's sake.

Monsanto and Lees, Mohawk and Dupont,
come in more colors if that's what you want.
Yet barefoottin's best in our turf heavensent,
though it's wise to beware of canine excrement.

Practically free, costs but a penny,
looking for faults, you'll find hardly any.
So don't be a crab - put it on the marquee!
What more could you want? I give up! What?  A tree?

So you hate ugly weeds and you don't like to mow,
and you don't like the early spring dandelion show.
Let's agree it's not perfect, but not quite so hasty,
'Cause if you're a cow, it's really quite tasty.

# Vacation

Time to plan that great vacation,
that most longed-for getaway,
far beyond the blue horizon,
Maybe Marakesh, Bombay.


You have a lot of comp time,
saved up from months of toil,
a week  to find a fair clime,
party hearty and uncoil.

A day to pack the haversack,
run the pup up to the kennel,
a day or two for travel
going intercontinental.


A day at least to acclimate
from lag and long layovers,
a day for the mandatory group tour
you'll take with your fellow rovers.

A day to moan upon the throne
from Montezuma's Revenge,
exotica's biotica
makes you wish for old Stonehenge.


Perhaps a day to pack things up,
(who knows what bargains you'll find),
A day to rest when you reach your nest,
a second time to unwind.


And - oops - I forgot, a day each way,
to visit remote kith and kin,
If my math is correct, I've got three hours to play,
So maybe I'll just sleep in.

## Hair

Let's talk about fuzzy, slick and unfair,
about straight, wavy, curly or not even there;
All shades of color in all kinds of places,
sheathing your bod or just  secretive spaces.

Short and long, thick and thin, all protein and pure,
but longer is better and more versus fewer.
Some people are bare where their hair used to sprout,
so they transplant, use Rogaine or just do without,

Women, I've noticed, soon have to renew it,
they style, wave and curl it; braid, twist and hue it.
No matter how beautiful soon comes the change -
like living room furniture - "Let's rearrange!"

Guys on the other hand, just leave it be,
till they can't hear or see, or use their ID.
Then off to the shop, where the barber goes wild,
"a bit off the top," and all's reconciled.

They want just  "a hair" of style, nothing too fussy,
so it looks good just hangin' there, even if mussy.
Most want it to look like it did yesterday;
some go into shock when it thins or turns gray.

# 8  The Smoking Poems

*Over the last fifteen years, our local hospital
has used various strategies to discourage smoking, a
laudable objective.  These poems reflect those strategies
and an observer's response.  They are in chronological order.
Personally, I do not smoke and do not advocate it.*

# The Smoking Atrium

Behold - our most cherished smoking retreat,
a place to inhale and yet be discreet,

the glass enclosure and central location
the choice of the hospital administration,

a few dying plants about to surrender
and nowhere in sight is the cigarette vendor,

air-conditioned year-round for your comfort or dis-
the puffers all shrouded in death-defying mist,

at night the incendiary sticks of the weed,
flit about like fire-flies feeding the need,

a kind of a habit becoming a yoke,
a kind of a cough becoming a choke,

taking your lungs and making a joke,
taking your money and leaving you broke.

One Hundred Feet


It's a really nasty habit with a price you'll have to pay,
This business of tobacco smoke is strictly declasse',
Secondhanders are at risk we know, no need to hold your breath,
Cause the powers that be have spoken, smokin' is the kiss of death.

If you have to cough or sneeze (thereby spreading some disease),
You can do it anytime or place and not disturb the peace,
But try to puff or drag near this place of getting well,
And they send out for security and bid you fond farewell,

A strange gray line surrounds the place from ashes on the ground
From smokers who are not yet wise just standing all around,
What have they got?  A parking lot! But stay out of the street!
A motley crew pass in review while trying to be discreet,

We wish them well, it's tough to see your friends be ostracized,
It's a habit or addiction as they define paradise,
The suggestion is to give it up, but "gee, it's tough" they say,
Compassion please, they're on their knees, one hundred feet away.

# Blowing Smoke

Closer now yet still outside the walls,
the inhalers take their modest pleasure alone
or in ever smaller groups.
Disdaining sweets and chews, and oblivious
of nicotine's grasp and carcinogen-laced cloud,
the world's greater bounty  seemingly out of reach,
blowing off the heavy haze of desperation,
rejecting the rejector's curtain of ostracizing edicts,
a few relaxing puffs on the weed
makes it all loom less large,
and more friendly like.

For some, a fair weather friend
beats no friend at all.

# 9    Perspectives of Pathos, Paradox and Passage

*When power narrows the areas of man's concern, poetry reminds him of the richness and diversity of his existence.  When power corrupts, poetry cleanses.*

John F. Kennedy

# Topical Anesthesia

Is it just the glow of the mesmerizing tube,
or the whole ball of wax,
Just the warm, barely compelling screen,
or the entire milieu of banality?

Electronic desensitization,
makes us numb and dumb,
less than we are,
or might become.

Tube effects can be temporary,
limited by the will,
switched off.

But fear the other,
society's *cool*,
coming from all sides,
taking the life away.

trax

From high above the pattern comes hard,
Chinese snowmobiles playing in the yard?
what they mean I'd like to know,
all those calligraphs in the snow.

pink slip


While you were out....
suddenly...
you're dismissed,
let go,
cast aside,
rendered obsolete,

(but what did I - why??)
just a reason,
(whatever... in a pig's eye)
not this season,

(time to pack)
when you're history
(can't get back - panic attack)
life's a mystery

(need to change?)
a little nosebleed
(Put it behind you, rearrange)
nothing's guaranteed

(Check your watch.)
Time to move on.
(Still top notch)
Begin and begone.

Experience


Yes, Virginia, you can catch lightning in a bottle.
But that doesn't mean it will stay there.
It won't - but you knew that.
At least you caught it once.
Some never do.

## The Fantasy

The fantasy has ended,
a dream in broken glass,
as crystalled dew in morning light
upon the new-mown grass,

Gone before the burning sun
will scorch the fragile earth,
vaporized without a trace
of all its joy at birth.

Engram


Push back  the memoried amazements,
force the daily automatics,
avoid, ignore,
search for the sense of it,
accept...

Work through the feelings,
wait for time's attrition,
skirt  the half-forgotten treasures,
the not-quite-out-of-reach traces of a
favorite song's salient strains,
a fire that raged,
a desolation...
wonder when the ash of memory
will disperse,
where it goes,
or if it goes at all,
or merely hides in a crease of convolutions,
only to reappear in cold three a m. sweat.

Moot

Gazing into your face,
your eyes locked on mine,
knowing, in sweet sadness,
no silly games
will ever be played,
that you see my soul too clearly
as I strain with yours;
it is not fair
you should be so sure of me,
while I wonder from microsecond to microsecond,
and pick the leaves from our four leaf clover.

## Shooting Stars

The dagger of morning light
slices  through  the  slit
twixt the shade and frame,
streaming across my bed.

Earth particles enter the beam,
f  l o a t   through,  and vanish.

Not as large, as fast or bright
as Perseids we never saw that
rainy August night in Jackson.

But I'm told their orbit is fixed,
even when receding, invisible
and almost forgotten,
and they always
come back,
for the
vu.

Druthers

There are only so many days of perfection,
days when the sun, the wind and the sky,
beckon the sailor like sirens of yore,
away from the land, away from the shore,
to spend on the water,
just one day more.

Such a day as today with the breeze ever soft,
I'd rather be watching my sails go aloft,
I'd rather consider the clouds on the fly,
I'd rather be sailing than wearing a tie.

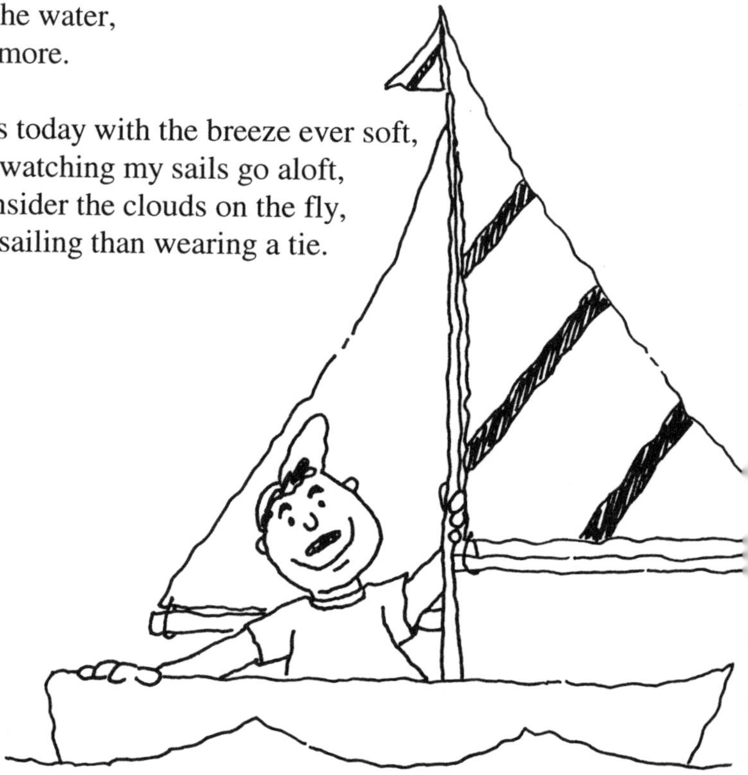

# ORDER FORM

Telephone Orders: Call Toll Free 1-800-247-6553
Have your VISA Mastercard, AMEX or Discover card ready.

Postal orders:  (CHECK OR MONEY ORDER ONLY)
Pantoum Press, P.O. Box 362, Painesville, OH 44077
Please send _________ copy/copies of "Topical Anesthesia"
at $11.95 per copy.
I understand that I may return any books for a full refund.

Name:_______________________________________________

Address:_____________________________________________

City:________________State________Zip_____________
Telephone: (_____)___________________
Sales Tax:
 Please add   $ 0.69 per copy for Ohio residents

Shipping and Handling:
    Book Rate: standard mail (3-4 weeks)  $2.00  first book, $.75
      ea. additional
    First Class: ( 2-10 days) $2.50  first book,  $1.50 ea. additional
    Priority Mail (2 days)  $4.00 first book, $3.50 ea. additional
Payment:
  _____Check
  _____Money Order